Spectacular Smiles, Superior Customer Service.

Today's Orthodontics

Bill M. Dischinger, DMD

To my wonderful family. My amazing wife and my remarkable boys, thank you for adventures!

I was fortunate to have an amazing mentor in my father, Terry Dischinger. I have had incredible teachers, colleagues and friends throughout my career that have taught me so much. My patients through the years have touched my life in so many ways. My team that I work with every day is the best in the orthodontic world. They make everyday in our office fun, rewarding and amazing. Thank you, thank you, thank you!

Contents

Introduction   9

Chapter 1 – Pain and Extractions and
             3 Years, Oh My!   11

Chapter 2 – Different Ways to Skin
             the Cat   19

Chapter 3 – Customer Service   25

Chapter 4 – Expanders and Self
             Ligating Braces   31

Chapter 5 - Esthetic Treatment for Adults
             (and kids for that matter)   43

Chapter 6 – I Want my Orthodontic
             Treatment Done Faster   47

Chapter 7 – Airway   53

Chapter 8 – Headaches   63

Chapter 9 – Orthodontics is Expensive   69

Conclusion   77

Spectacular Smiles, Superior Customer Service.

Today's Orthodontics

Introduction

Orthodontics requires teeth to be pulled. Expanders are necessary to widen the jaws. Treatment will take 2 years. Orthodontics is painful. Orthodontics is only for kids and can only be done correctly with braces. Orthodontic treatment is expensive and not very affordable. These statements are all myths. In today's world they just are not true. There are a few exceptions, but in today's orthodontic office these statements should all be false for virtually every patient.

Orthodontics, just like the world around us, has evolved greatly over the last decade. This short and easy read is intended to help individuals and families that are looking into orthodontics be better educated and capable of making the best decisions for their orthodontic treatment. Let's dive in and learn some things together!

Chapter 1

Pain and Extractions and 3 Years, Oh My!

Other than cost, the main questions every patient asks are:

- How much will this hurt?

- Do I need to have teeth pulled?

- How long is this going to take?

In this book these questions will be answered. As an adult, most of us remember our orthodontic experience not as a fun and fond memory, but in varying degrees of negativity to these 3 questions. Thankfully for anyone having treatment today, orthodontics is no longer like walking to school in the snow, uphill both ways. Braces have historically been viewed in the same light as having a colonoscopy: a necessary evil in life. Although the resulting beautiful smile was "worth it in the end," wouldn't it be great if the process was not like training for an ironman triathlon? "I'm so glad I did it, but I couldn't go through that again."

Why was orthodontics of the past so much more difficult than today? Why is orthodontics today so much less painful and long than in the past? The answer is technology and the super smart people that advanced it along the way!

Technology has changed everything in our lives. When I was growing up, we had 5 channel, including the public broadcasting channel which was pretty much worthless after Sesame Street ended each morning. Today's TV world is so overwhelming in its choices that at times, the entertainment is just scrolling through the channels to see what we are missing rather than actually watching shows.

Cassette tapes? Remember sitting with your finger hovering over the "play/record" button, waiting for that song to come on the radio? You knew things were getting serious when you received that "mixed tape". Thanks to Steve Jobs and the iPod, now even CDs are obsolete. And then there is the greatest invention in the history of man. The car? No. Airplanes? No. American Football? Almost. The smart phone. How in the world did we survive before cell phones, let alone smart phones? Just the maps feature alone has saved many a marriage. "Honey, let's just stop and ask for directions". "Dear, I know where we are," without Siri, 30 minutes have passed and they are still not at their destination and all conversation has stopped. If they are talking, Honey and Dear are long gone.

The first year I had my iPhone, I didn't know there was more than the first home page. When I discovered that side swipe to get to page 2, I thought, "Why would I ever need that many apps?" Now I'm 10 pages deep and counting.

These examples of technology have changed our lives forever, but only if we embrace them. They all had a learning curve with some frustration along the way. All new technology does. Orthodontics is no different. The first great invention in orthodontics came in the form of a chemistry breakthrough: Adhesives. My early memories of braces was the classic "railroad tracks" look. Orthodontists used to have to put a band (or ring) around each tooth to secure the brace to it. This was quite the "joyful" experience. Orthodontist: "I'm going to lightly tap on this band to place it around your tooth." "Bang, bang, bang!" At this point you were usually hovering somewhere between horror and passing out.

By the 1970's new technology in the world of adhesives had found its way into orthodontics. It allowed orthodontists to glue a brace onto the front of the tooth rather than use all those bands. The advantages of this process were many. One of the biggest advantages of not having all the extra metal of bands in between the teeth was that more cases could be treated without the extraction of teeth.

Later that decade, an amazingly brilliant orthodontist named Larry Andrews invented the straight wire appliance. Historically, braces were a way to grab a hold of the tooth. The orthodontist would use a series of stainless steel wires that he/she put various bends into to straighten the teeth. The wire provided all the angles, bends, tips, etc. to properly align the teeth. The braces were just the means to attach the wire to the teeth. Dr. Andrews changed that. He built braces that had all these angles, tips, etc. built into them. Each tooth in the mouth had a specific brace, with its own set of movements preprogrammed into it. This allowed the orthodontist to place the wire into the braces and the teeth would get pretty close to where they were supposed to be. The orthodontist would then just need to make minor adjustments in the last wires to get those final details done. This shortened treatment times and helped make visits to the office less frequent and slightly less painful. It also made the job much easier for orthodontists; allowing them to delegate more of the work to dental assistants. By doing this, orthodontists could treat more patients in a day, allowing them to keep the cost of orthodontics affordable. The inflation of orthodontic treatment over the past 40 years is miniscule compared to the actual inflation rate; in particular the inflation rate within the medical world.

Around the same time that Dr. Andrews invented the straight wire appliance, the world of orthodontics borrowed some technology from NASA. The space shuttle was where they tested many metal combinations. From these tests came the perfect blend to go along with Dr. Andrews' braces. Nickel and titanium. When blended together, these wires can be shaped into a perfect mouth arch form. The beauty in these wires is that they retain their shape after being distorted, bent and twisted. This means that when put in a mouth of crooked teeth, the wire slowly straightens back out to its original shape, thus straightening the teeth. No longer did orthodontists have to keep putting in stainless steel wires that continually were deformed. Appointments could be spread farther apart as adjustments didn't need to occur as frequently. The wires also delivered less force to the teeth, which we will learn in chapter 4 is very important. Orthodontics, like the world around us, has greatly changed with the technology advancements of the past 40 years.

Chapter 2

Different Ways to Skin the Cat

"We have been to 3 orthodontic offices and they all have a different plan. We are totally confused." I hear this in my office every week. How can the same mouth have such different plans to correct it? Well, orthodontics is as much an art as it is science. We are working in the field of perception. Beauty is in the eye of the beholder, right? Well, orthodontic results and more to this point, orthodontic treatments, are in the hands of the beholder.

I grew up in a basketball family. My father played on the 1960 Olympic Gold medal basketball team with legends such as Oscar Robertson and Jerry West. He was Rookie of the Year in the 1962-63 NBA season. I have seen a lot of basketball in my life and thus, I've seen many players shoot a basketball. There is no one way to shoot. Many ways work. Lots of different forms can get the ball into the hoop. Similarly, many ways of orthodontics can get teeth straight as well.

I chose a specific method that works very well in my hands, but I also feel makes a lot of sense from a health perspective as well. We'll discuss this system in chapter 4.

Remember when I said beauty is in the eye of the beholder? Beauty, though, is not just straight teeth. In my opinion, the best orthodontists in the world treat much more than just teeth. We treat faces! What good is it for me to straighten out teeth if I totally disregard the position, size and shape of your lips? Of your chin? Of your cheeks and nose? Where your teeth fit in your smile? Whether you show more gum tissue than normal? When orthodontics is done properly, it takes into account all of those aspects of aesthetics. Facial balance and smile aesthetics drive all my decisions of how best to treat my patients. Straightening the teeth is easy. Facial aesthetics is where the beauty of our art comes into play. Have you ever seen a person that finished braces and it looked like their lips had gotten smaller? How about a finished treatment where the upper front teeth were all flat, straight across and looked like fake denture teeth; or a person whose chin was weak or too far back? These are all examples of aesthetic orthodontic failures. Great orthodontic treatment will result in facial balance and smile harmony, not just a set of straight teeth.

The upper teeth should have a curve to them that follows the natural curve of the lower lip when smiling. Get up and go to a mirror. Smile in the mirror. Do your teeth have that natural curve to them that matches the curve of your smiling lower lip? If not, we can change that.

In our office, we push ourselves to be on the cutting edge of treatments for people that have a lower jaw that didn't grow as much as it should and for patients with a weak chin even developing the appliance that corrects that problem. It is called the AdvanSync, although many know it as the Herbst. I've been honored to give over 100 lectures in the U.S and around the world on this and other techniques. We are able to use this appliance to move an underdeveloped lower jaw forward to give facial balance and a stronger chin.

Orthodontics in today's world is for more than just straightening some teeth. A great orthodontist will look at every aspect of your facial aesthetics. If they're not, it would be like passing up a new smart phone in favor of an old flip phone. You can still make phone calls, but you're missing a whole other world.

Chapter 3

Customer Service

My story:

Growing up, my plan was to play basketball.

As mentioned earlier, I grew up with a father that played in the NBA. Following his career, he became an orthodontist. As a kid, I naturally assumed I would be in the NBA. Somehow the basketball world overlooked my talent and I had to make other career plans.

My introduction to the orthodontic world came the summer after my freshman year in college. I didn't have my summer job lined up yet and my dad needed somebody to fill in a position in his lab at the office. It didn't take me long to see what a great profession this was. People's lives were transformed on a daily basis. You may doubt that, but research shows that people with nice smiles have better jobs, are better liked and feel better about themselves. It's unfortunate this the world that we live in, where judgments are made based on how a person looks, but it's true. I saw that orthodontics could impact lives in a way few other professions can. But it was more than that. The office had an environment that I'd never seen anywhere else. Every person on the team had one focus; one purpose: to deliver the best customer service experience possible to every person who passed through the door. Patients and parents were genuinely excited to be there. I decided that summer I would be an orthodontist. I loved everything about it.

Unfortunately, in today's world a great customer service experience is few and far between.

Heck, even avoiding bad customer service experiences is hard to do. My dad used to say: "We have no idea what is going on in their life or how their day has been going. Their best experience of the day will be when they come into our office and we will have an impact on their life." What a great way to run a business! He passed that mindset on to me and our team has continued to live by that mindset.

Isn't it easier and more rewarding to go through the day having fun and being nice to people? It just seems so natural to me. It takes a lot of energy to be grumpy and angry. When I drive on our roads and people give me that special "peace" sign, I just laugh. It would be sad to go through life like that.

Our goal as a team is to make every experience in our office the best experience of the day for our patients and parents. Of the week. Just the best, period.

It starts with a mindset. It then turns into a culture. I'm a bit of a Disney Geek. I love going to the parks for many reasons, but one of the biggest is their level of customer service. They call it the Disney Experience and many books and training programs have come out of it. In fact, we once took one of the training programs as a team. What I love is that if you ask a question of a "cast member", they all either know the answer, or if they don't, they point you to who you should talk to. They personally will walk you to that person. The attention to detail in every aspect of the park, especially when it comes to customer service and communication, is the best in the world.

That's how an orthodontic office should be. It shouldn't be the sliding glass window at the front desk that we get at our doctor's office. It should literally be like going to Disneyland! The customer service experience should not be limited to the patient. It should extend to the entire family. That may be letting the younger siblings watch their older brother or sister get their braces on or being able to take part in the prizes and games at the appointments. Moms and Dads should be pampered while their child is being treated as well. Our lives are so busy. Isn't it nice to be able to sit down and take a breath? Have a seat in a massage chair, have a paraffin hand treatment and enjoy some refreshments. Let your kids be entertained with some video games, iPads or movies. Take a break. We want every member of the family to look forward to coming to our office. We want it to be a highlight within your hectic life.

We all remember bad experiences, but you know, we remember those extraordinary ones even more vividly. That's the way customer service ought to be.

Chapter 4

Expanders and Self Ligating Braces

"I went to an orthodontist and they told me my child needs a palatal expander." Many times when we are a second opinion on treatment, we hear this. For the first 5-6 years of my orthodontic career, I used expanders on a very large percentage of my young patients. Around 2005 though, some research began to surface about some of the negative side effects that can occur after expander use; the main concern was that in some cases the molar hooked to by the expander would get pushed out of the bone and not heal properly. Long term, this would lead to gum and bone problems, which require gum grafts or other procedures as an adult to correct. This does not occur in a majority of patients, but how would you feel if you were on the operating table getting ready for heart surgery, and the surgeon told you "Most of the time this goes great, but 25% of my patients die during this." I'd jump off the table. Thankfully, orthodontics is not life or death, but we'd still like to avoid causing damage as we perform the orthodontics.

I decided I needed to find a different way to widen my dental arches and make room for the teeth. This began my journey into seeing how effectively light-force orthodontics can change our mouths. We will learn what light force orthodontics is in the coming pages.

While at my residency at Tufts University in Boston, I heard a remarkable lecture by a brilliant orthodontist from Spokane, Washington. His name was Dwight Damon and he had invented a brace system called the Damon System (not very originally named, I know). Since the 1940's, braces had the wires held in place by little stainless steel wires secured around each brace. In the 1980's the color ties were invented (you know, all the colors the kids have on their braces?). Where technology was at the time, these were the only ways to hold the wire in place, and this didn't change for almost 60 years! Dr. Damon changed that though. His brace had a little door that opened, the wire was put into the brace (just like other braces) but then the door was closed, keeping the wire in the brace. OK, what's the big deal? Well for that, unfortunately I'm going to have to first give you a physics lesson, followed by a biography lesson. I promise it will be way more fun than reading your old high school science books. Let's start with Physics. My wife loves to make me move our furniture around. Before my boys were old enough and strong enough to help me, I had to do it all by myself. One day at Home Depot, I saw this thing called Furniture Caddy. It consisted of these little coasters that you would put under each leg of the furniture piece. I know many of you are nodding your heads right now because you have them, too. When you put these in place, you could literally push the furniture with one finger. Why though? Friction. By putting these smooth, plastic discs under the feet, it gave a smooth, slick surface that easily slides on the floor. It greatly reduced the friction that was normally being generated between the contact of the furniture foot with the floor. It's like you threw a layer of grease on the floor. It's so cool! (Yes, I'm a science geek). Yeah, so that relates to teeth how? Remember those ties that held the wire in place? They held it in place very tightly. By doing that, it's like putting a bungee cord around the brace and wire. For the wire to move, it has to overcome all the friction generated by that tie against the wire. Well again, why does that matter? Well, to move any tooth, the wire has to slide through all the braces on the teeth behind that crooked tooth. Let's look at a pretty easy example and help illustrate this. Have you ever seen someone with their upper canine tooth (some people call it an eye tooth) stuck up high? It looks like a fang. When we attach the brace to that tooth to bring it down into place, we have to take the wire and snake it up high, bending it quite a bit and then back down again to the brace behind it. As that tooth comes down, all that extra wire that was used to go up to the tooth has to slide through the other braces. We want it to slide through those back braces. If it can't slide through the back braces, it slides forward. Unfortunately this causes the front teeth to be pushed or flared forward. That's not a good thing and results in a "bucked tooth" smile. To combat that, the orthodontist needed to extract teeth in order to pull those front teeth backwards into the extraction spaces and counteract this movement. This is another reason there has been a high rate of extracting historically. If we have those ties on the wires and braces, the friction is high and the wire can't slide (just like my furniture without the caddies) towards the back, and the front teeth flare forward. That's problem number one with those ties.

Problem number two is that to overcome that friction to just actually move a tooth, aside from worrying about flaring the teeth forward, we had to push really hard on them. Just like me getting a full workout when pushing the furniture without the coasters. What do you think happens to our teeth when we push on them? Inflammation, and then the teeth hurt. Inflammation is not a good thing. We want to minimize inflammation as much as we can. When inflammation occurs, the teeth don't move as efficiently because the body reacts first in a negative way. So, to minimize inflammation, we push more gently on the teeth.

During first week of my orthodontic residency program in Boston, I read the 2nd chapter in my text book. A doctor named Carl Sandstedt in 1926 said that we should only push on the teeth with a maximum of 26 grams of force. This is because when blood flows through the capillaries, that is how much force it pushes outward against the walls of the vessel. If the force is above that, the wall collapses and blood no longer can flow to the tissues around the tooth. When this happens, oxygen can't get to the cells that cause the bone to change to allow the tooth to move. Okay Carl, got it. 26 grams of force. Now on to Chapter 3: Orthodontic wires. It said, "Orthodontic wires exert a force of 60-120 grams of force. These are the fundamental working wires of orthodontics." What? Wait a minute. Carl told us to not go above 26 grams. Is there something I'm missing? Is it in chapter 4? Nope, it wasn't. There was no explanation, because the technology needed to use forces as low as Carl had told us to use had not been invented yet. Our brace systems had too much friction to let us use forces that low. The wire couldn't move. It couldn't overcome the friction. It got stuck unless the force was increased to beat the friction. Our systems were flawed. But nobody talked about it until Dr. Damon. His system eliminated friction. Now, all we had to do was overcome the biological force needed to move a tooth. We could use way lighter wires to move teeth. We could do what Dr. Carl had told us to do. We were now moving teeth in a biologically appropriate manner. We were working with the body rather than against it. The body is amazing. If you guide it, it responds. If you hammer it, it rebels. Hammering is what we used to do in orthodontics. There is an old joke: "How does the orthodontist know what size wire to put in my braces?" The assistant answers, "When he can feel your heart beat through your teeth, he knows he's got the right one." Seriously, that is how it used to be. I used to look at a tooth and the brace on it and figure how I could place the biggest, boldest wire in there. I wanted to hammer on that tooth as hard as I could to overcome my brace technology. Now I can decide what is the lightest force I can use to accomplish my objective. A completely different mindset from what I had prior to seeing this technology. This now allows us to gently push or guide the teeth where we want them to go. I can get the bone to adapt and change in ways we never could before the Damon System. I no longer need that palatal expander to widen the upper jaw. The bone will now widen as it is guided to do so with the light forces. Dr. Damon completely opened my eyes to how I could treat patients. It took me over 6 years to fully realize and master this concept, but now I am able to treat the body in a healthy, more naturalistic way. You may be asking, "Why doesn't everyone use this method, then?" Well, I don't know, but when change is made it takes time. If I knew the answer to helping make change easy, I could write another book that cures obesity, smoking, alcoholism and probably even divorce.

As I stated, it took me 6 years to master this technique and most of us aren't willing or patient enough to go through a learning curve such as that. There are orthodontists that continue to use traditional braces with 40 year old technology, and state that Damon braces, or braces similar to them don't matter; that is fine for them, they are entitled to their opinion. But let me ask you this. What would you rather have pushing on your teeth? Heavy forces that cause high inflammation or light forces that gently move the teeth with minimal inflammation? I know, me too!

Chapter 5

Esthetic Treatment for Adults (and kids for that matter)

More and more adults are seeking orthodontic treatment to help create the smile they have always dreamed of. Fortunately, we are keeping our teeth our entire life in today's dental world, and many adults want them to look their best. Not only is a smile important for adults, but the bite is even more important. Now that we are not losing our teeth to decay and disease, they must be protected from harm. If a bite is off, the teeth may eventually crack, wear down or notch at the gumline along with risking gum recession. Due to all these reasons, more and more adults are seeking orthodontic treatment. One of the first concerns is if they will have a mouth full of metal? The answer is no! There are cosmetic or clear options available. Clear braces are no longer those ugly, yellow, stained bubbles that look like popcorn stuck on your teeth. In our office, we use the best clear brace available, made of a polycrystalline that is truly clear, so it basically dissolves into the natural color of the teeth. And they work! Possibly the most popular treatment (at least the most asked about) is Invisalign. While I took the first Invisalign Training course offered in the northwest back in 1999, very few of the early cases I treated with it turned out right. Fast forward to today and it's much different. It is now a very good product. It still can't treat everything, but it can treat a lot, and very well.

Invisalign did an amazing job marketing itself and virtually everyone has heard of it. It has allowed people that have a fear of wearing braces (particularly adults) to now undergo orthodontic treatment and obtain that smile they've dreamed of. What a gift! Invisalign can be more expensive than braces in many cases, as it is the most expensive product for orthodontists to use, but for many patients, it is worth it.

Another advantage of Invisalign is for patients with metal allergies. Most metal braces and wires contain nickel, which ironically, is the most common metal allergy. For patients with nickel allergies, Invisalign has provided us with an avenue to treat them in a healthy, sustainable way.

Chapter 6

I Want My Orthodontic Treatment Done Faster

I have to say, in all my years as an orthodontist, I've only met about 2-3 patients that didn't desire this. As I mentioned earlier in the book, "How long will my treatment take?" is one of the first questions asked.

This has become increasingly more important as our society, our entire world, has become the "now" generation. Everything is right at our fingertips immediately. At the time of writing this book, Amazon has recently launched its 1-hour delivery. Seriously! That's crazy! I don't have to go to a store, and I don't have to wait days for it to arrive? Sign me up! What if we could speed up the whole orthodontic process and shorten our treatment times? Again, sign me up!

Remember in our earlier chapter reading about the light forces we now use with orthodontic treatment? That alone speeds up the rate of tooth movement for the physiological reasons discussed. The same thing can also be done with Invisalign treatment too by doing less movement per aligner but changing the aligners twice as fast. This again lowers the forces; the teeth move faster and you can progress through the overall treatment faster.

There are a few other ways of shortening the length of treatment. These involve additional procedures or devices added to the treatment plan.

For many years there has been a technique available that introduces trauma to the bone, which causes the rate of bone healing or change to occur faster. It is quite involved and is done outside the orthodontists' office. A dental surgical specialist makes cuts in the bone after temporarily pulling back the gum tissue. This trauma increases the amount of blood flow to the area, leading to an increase of bone change rate, thus faster tooth movement. Okay, hopefully we've all recovered from fainting now and we are ready to hear of a better way to do this.

More recently, this process has been simplified and now is done much easier in the orthodontic office. Some simple local numbing is done and then we orthodontists actually use a little pin to "punch" holes into the bone, creating a similar response to the scary procedure talked about above. For sure, this may still sound scary, but I can tell you, its actually quite easy. The drawback, though, is that it has to be done twice during treatment as the effects only last for 6 months. Still feeling a bit light headed? Well, there are two other techniques, both of which are not invasive.

A brand-new technique uses a specialized type of light that produces what is called a photo modulation response at a cellular level. Basically, the cells make more energy and can work faster at changing the bone to allow tooth movement. It's pretty exciting, but at this point in time, fairly expensive. The take home units are over $1,000 USD.

The most common type of tooth acceleration technique being used today are micro pulsation units. For many years, orthopedic surgeons have used this technique to aid in bone fracture healing. In 2012 the technique was approved for orthodontics. The patient is given a mouthpiece that attaches to a small, rechargeable unit that delivers these micro-pulses to the teeth. It is used every day for 5 to 20 minutes depending on the frequency level used. For Invisalign treatments, it allows us to change the aligners twice as fast (each aligner is worn for half the normal amount of time), thus reducing treatment time by 50%. For braces, I am seeing about a 25% reduction in time using this device. We can now treat pretty much any Invisalign case in under one year.

Reduced treatment time is not the only benefit, though. The process lowers the amount of inflammation that occurs during tooth movement, which thus lowers the level of pain. Typically, orthodontics can at times hurt at about a 5 on a 1-10 pain scale. Using this technology brings this down to a 1 or 2 for both braces and Invisalign. These micropulse devices typically add an additional $350-$500

to a patient's treatment. This cost will most likely

continue to go down.

Chapter 7

Airway

If you're like me, while in the car, you listen to the radio. The stations I listen to promote retainers to wear at night to stop snoring. I guess that shows the demographics of the stations I listen to (I never thought I'd be as old as my parents). Why is snoring such a big deal now? We've all spent vacations with our grandparents, and grandpa always snored. Grandma sometimes did too. Well, in medicine they have discovered this actually isn't a normal part of getting old, but a sign of what's called sleep apnea. Sleep apnea has become the "buzz phrase" lately in medicine. It's very obvious in adults, particularly in males. They typically appear to stop snoring for 5-20 seconds, then take a big snort or snore and start breathing again. We used to think this was just snoring loudly or strongly. We now know they actually stop breathing and their oxygen levels drop. This is quite common in adults, particularly men, but did you know that it is quite prevalent in children, too? We shouldn't hear kids breathing as they sleep. Most kids with airway issues don't snore as we would typically describe it. It's usually more like a loud breathing.

Studies state that 10% of children are described as having sleep apnea. This is the actual diagnosed level by pediatricians. I can tell you this is vastly underestimated though. How many of you have had your pediatrician ask you if Johnny or Suzi snore? Probably few of you at best. Pediatricians unfortunately just don't have the time to discuss every single issue that could be going on. They have to look for the "bad" stuff. But did you know that over

25% of kids that are diagnosed with ADHD actually don't have it? They just don't get proper sleep due to airway issues. These can then manifest themselves in ways such as ADHD (or just daytime fidgetiness), morning and evening tiredness and over activeness. So many of our little boys have this issue, but have been "labeled" in school as boys that can't pay attention. It happens in girls as well, but many of the girls are able to overcome the ADHD behavior better than boys and not receive this label.

So what causes these airway issues and how do we change it? Airway issues could be caused by one or many things at once. The one we all probably know about is enlarged tonsils. In the 60's – 80's, taking out tonsils was quite common. Remember Peter Brady on the Brady Bunch? Then there was a huge swing the other way where it was hardly ever done. Now we are starting to swing a little back up as airway issues are being more recognized. In most cases, the adenoids are also a problem when the tonsils become enlarged. Adenoids are located farther back and up the throat than tonsils and can only be seen through imaging techniques. If one or both of these are enlarged, the airway is greatly compromised and should be removed. My youngest son had this procedure done and his airway improved significantly.

Nasal obstructions can occur as well. Yes, sometimes when someone has that deviated septum repaired, they actually are telling the truth and didn't have a nose job. The turbinates' in the nasal cavity sometimes need to be reshaped as well.

That's all great, but why am I talking about airway in a book that's supposed to be about orthodontics?

Well, it is very easy for orthodontists that own a certain type of x-ray machine to evaluate the airway. There is a new x-ray machine called CBCT. Stands for Cone Beam Computed Tomography. Basically, it takes a 3 dimensional x-ray with Cat-Scan ability to see the soft tissue. It can give the exact measurement of a person's airway volume. The machine takes about 8 seconds to take a scan with a dosage of 17 micro sieverts. The American Radiology Board recommends we keep our radiation exposure below 1,000 micro sieverts per year. Pretty amazing machine, huh? We take one of these scans on all our patients, and airway evaluation is part of the diagnosis. Many patients with airway issues will have a poor position of their tongue. Our tongue is supposed to rest in the roof of our mouth and when we swallow, it should slightly touch the back of our front teeth up near the gumline. Yes, I can see you swallowing and thinking about it right now. A lot of people have a narrow palate, and the tongue is unable to do this. It sits low and farther back, the last contributor in causing a blockage of the airway.

Remember discussing jaws that are positioned too far back? The lower jaw is the most common and biggest contributor, but sometimes the upper jaw can be at fault, too. So, your orthodontist should be looking at this as part of their routine evaluations.

What can we do though? Many things! First, if tonsils or adenoids are issues, I will refer you to an ENT to have them evaluated and possibly removed. If the palate is narrow, we can widen and enlarge it to its proper dimension. As discussed earlier, we can do this with our light force braces. There are some situations though, that I would use a palatal expander. Wait, you thought I said I don't use palatal expanders? Well, this is one time I would. Sometimes. Okay, now you're really confused. Let me explain. Sometimes I will have a child come in that has very severe airway issues, and it has greatly affected their ability to behave properly or even not wet the bed. If I use my light force braces, I will change this, but it will take 6-8 months to see a change in these side effects. If we use a palatal expander, we'll see results in 2-4 weeks. We attach the expander onto the baby teeth, not the permanent molars, so we won't see any long term problems with these teeth. When the palate is widened to its proper size, the airway will increase significantly, and most times to its proper volume. For these kids that have an airway issue that affects their success in school, they just can't wait for me to take 6-8 months to help them. They need help now. These are the kids I will use an expander on.

If the mandible (lower jaw) is too far back, we use our AdvanSync appliance I already discussed in chapter 2 to correct it. This change will greatly increase the airway volume as well.

The last issue is the upper jaw being too far back. This is something that will result in an Underbite (the lower front teeth biting forward of the upper front teeth). This would be the other time I use a palatal expander because research has shown that the use of an expander aids in the forward movement of the upper jaw when used with an appliance that helps it come forward.

Let's review what signs to look for in your children if you suspect an airway issue. Snoring or loud breathing while sleeping (or even while awake for that matter). And for heaven's sake, if they are actually stopping breathing, take them straight to an orthodontist that can take a CBCT scan or to an ENT today! If you can actually see their tonsils when they open, they are enlarged. They will be these big red balls that puff out towards the middle of the throat when they open wide. You can actually see them move towards the middle as they say "Ah". ADHD behavior can be due to airway issues, and is suspected to be the true culprit in 25% of children with an ADHD diagnosis. Lastly, one we haven't talked about. If your child grinds their teeth at night, they have an airway issue. This is the brain trying to move the jaw around in an attempt to open up that airway.

Pediatric airway issues are a huge epidemic in our society that, unfortunately, are being overlooked by the medical world. In orthodontics, particularly in an office that understands airway issues, this can and must change!

Chapter 8

Headaches

Headaches? Why is an orthodontist writing about headaches? That's exactly what I would have thought prior to 2014. But then I was exposed to a product that's sole purpose was to help patients dealing with chronic pain, specifically headaches. Are any of you migraine sufferers? I used to fall into this group. Fortunately, some minor orthodontic fine tuning and some simple dietary modification facilitated by my naturopath have helped. Occasionally, though, I will still get one. Almost always these are the result of an extended period of lack of sleep and stress. On the very rare times these hit me, the treatments we now have in my office give me a non-drug solution.

Let's first discuss what causes headaches, what a headache is, and how the whole head plays into them.

The World Health Organization estimates that 12% of Americans suffer from migraines. A large group of this 12% have been unsuccessful in finding treatments that help them and are chronic pain suffers. 80% of migraines are caused by an issue in the oral cavity or muscles of the jaw and neck. The majority of pain nerves in the face, neck and jaws all converge into one place called the Trigeminal Nucleus. It's kind of like the fuse box of our head. Pretty much, almost all head pain is transmitted, altered or modified through the Trigeminal Nucleus.

The product I mentioned earlier is called TruDenta. It is a system that thoroughly analyzes the whole head and neck complex of a patient. This includes a full health history, muscle palpitation, TMJ assessment, Dental assessment including a force analysis and a range of motion analysis. Through all of this analysis, we identify the problem areas. These areas are being transmitted through the Trigeminal Nucleus, which in turn leads to referred pain in other areas, typically headaches, or worse, migraines. The TruDenta System has a 93% success rate in providing patients with real, long lasting relief from their pain symptoms. The system includes 4 areas of treatment. These are:

1. Muscle and soft tissue rehabilitation

   a) In office therapy

   b) Ultrasound

   c) Manual manipulation (massage)

   d) Micro current

e) Cold laser therapy

2. TMD treatment

   a) Oral appliances

   b) Short term medication, if needed

   c) Exercise

3. Bite imbalances

   a) Dental disease treatment, if needed

   b) Bite force balancing

   c) Orthodontic treatment, if needed

   d) New dental restorations, if needed

4. Home care program

   a) Stretching and exercises

   b) Natural anti-inflammatories

c) Psychological stress management, if needed

d) Sleep management as needed.

So, back to the original question: Why an orthodontist? We are the only healthcare practitioners that can work both inside and outside the mouth. Just like medical doctors, we have extensive fundamental medical training in anatomy and physiology, with particular emphasis on the head and neck. We can prescribe x-rays, use physical therapy, massage, intramuscular stimulation, sport rehabilitation techniques and devices inside the mouth, all within one office by one practitioner. Most importantly, the diagnosis and treatment of 80% of the pain found in the head and neck region falls within the scope of dental and orthodontic practices.

To summarize our chapter on headaches and migraines: pain (typically headache/migraine) is caused by instability or imbalance of the teeth, muscles or both. These cause pain that is transmitted, altered or modified by the Trigeminal Nucleus. Orthodontists are the best healthcare provider to assess and treat this type of symptom in the head and neck areas because this is the world we work in all day, every day. Treatments will include rehabilitative therapy outside the mouth and, in most cases, inside the mouth as well. The great news is that with the TruDenta System, 93% of patients have a dramatic reduction, if not complete elimination, in the frequency, intensity and duration of chronic pain.

Chapter 9

Orthodontics is Expensive!

Orthodontics is not affordable! Remember early in the book we said there were some myths about orthodontics out there? This is one of them. I feel helping with the cost of a college education is the best use of our money for our children. The second best is investing in a beautiful smile for them. I am, of course, biased with my opinion because of what I do for a living, but as we mentioned, research shows how important an attractive smile is in our societies. Given that I feel this strongly about orthodontic treatment, I decided to write a chapter to help families learn and know more to make treatment more affordable.

Many companies offer programs for their employees called Flexible Spending Accounts or Health Savings Accounts. Using these accounts to pay for treatment allows you to use pre-tax dollars for treatment. Many Flexible Spending Accounts let you put up to $2500/year toward qualified health care expenses, which include orthodontics. With Health Savings Accounts, you may be able to pay for the entire treatment, pre-taxed. Using these accounts creates a significant tax advantage and can be the most powerful way to save money on your orthodontic treatment. Make sure you pay attention to your company deadlines if you plan to use flex spending dollars. Most companies require you to let them know ahead of time if you plan to use flex dollars and how much you would like to save into an account. Check with your specific company, but most companies have either November or June enrollment periods. Failing to sign up in time could cost you significantly more out-of-pocket dollars to pay for your treatment. Most orthodontists offer free consultations, so be sure to get an orthodontic exam before the deadline to register for your flex account.

If you have orthodontic insurance, congratulations! Approximately 50% of those seeking orthodontic treatment do not have the ability to take advantage of insurance benefits.

Make sure to check with your employer as to what type of insurance is available to you. Many have different options for orthodontic coverage. Some insurances also now require a one-year waiting period. So, you may have to sign up now for benefits next year. If you, or a family member, may be interested in orthodontics in the future, check with your insurance supplier to make sure you get the most benefit from your insurance. Also, a common misconception is that you can only see an in-network orthodontist. FALSE! For almost all orthodontic insurances, you will still get the same insurance benefit regardless of if you see an in-network doctor or not. When you visit an orthodontist, they should provide you with a complimentary insurance benefits check.

Most offices will offer you several options to pay for treatment. Typically, you can pay for treatment in full and save a percentage on treatment, you can use a down payment and break payments into 1-2 years of monthly payments, or you can opt for an extended financing plan. If you choose an extended financing plan, watch for hidden fees or surprise charges if you miss a payment. You shouldn't need to pay higher than 10% APR for an extended (over 24 month) payment plan. You should also have the option for shorter payment plans to have 0% APR. Companies like OrthoFi are helping doctors make treatment more and more affordable for patients by giving them many different options to customize paying for treatment.

When comparing the price for orthodontists, look closely at the cheapest price. Many offices offer low prices up front, but hit you with many fees later in treatment which can make the total cost for treatment much higher. Broken bracket fees, missed appointment fees, cancellation fees, not including retainers in the overall price, separate fees for x-rays, etc. These can dramatically increase the total cost of treatment. Beware of any office that charges additional monthly fees after a certain point. For example, many offices can start charging extra if treatment extends beyond 24 months. This actually creates an incentive for the office to keep your braces on longer so that the office can charge more. Also, lower-cost offices typically use lower-cost materials. Braces can be purchased from third-world manufacturers for a fraction of the cost of American-made braces. But, all braces are not created equal. Using a cheaper brace often leads to months or years longer in braces and 10 or 15 additional visits during treatment. Would you pay a few hundred dollars extra to be done with your braces sooner and to have many less trips into the office for adjustments? Consider this before selecting your orthodontist. Shopping for the cheapest orthodontic treatment in town may come with a significant cost; in dollars, in your time, and in your comfort.

We know that orthodontic treatment is a financial investment and for many families, this is a significant financial decision. We have talked about what a difference orthodontic treatment can make in a person's life. Our goal is for everyone that seeks treatment at our office to be able to afford it. We have partnered with OrthoFi, a company mentioned earlier. With their help, we have seen finances be removed as a barrier to starting treatment with us. I definitely encourage you to work with an office that is willing to work with you financially so that orthodontics is not a burden financially, but something that can fit within your family's budget.

Conclusion

Time to wake back up, you've reached the end of the book. If you made it this far, you deserve a prize. You won't get a prize, but you deserve one.

Thank you for coming along with me on an orthodontic learning ride. Today's orthodontics is light years ahead of where it once was. A beautiful, well balanced face and smile is attainable, more comfortable, faster and affordable. Take that next step and call an orthodontist near you. If you live in the Pacific Northwest, we'd love to see you in our office. You're just a phone call away from a Spectacular Smile with Superior Customer Service!